Shingles Relief!
Cutting Through the BS
What Works. What Doesn't

by
Alan Novarc

Cover Design: Louise Guibesi

ISBN 978-1-365-34264-6

10 9 8 7 6 5 4 3 2

Printed in the USA

About the author

Despite satisfying the course and grade requirements for application to medical school, the author finished up with a university degree in anthropology, an area of life-long interest. Cultural notions of health and wellbeing have been a consistent source of fascination over the past 25 years, especially local pharmacopeias and notions of mind/body interrelationships.

Dedication

To practitioners everywhere
who passionately embrace the healing arts

Contents

Preface

In some of its iterations, shingles can be a dangerous disease. Especially in cases where the eye or eyes are involved, it is very important to seek treatment immediately. In all cases, the quickest possible intervention is important in order to reduce the possibility of resulting post-herpetic neuralgia (PHN). Do not underestimate the extent to which PHN can reduce quality of life. PHN is a leading contributing factor to the decision to commit suicide among the elderly.

Introduction

Probably since the beginning of time, whenever there's been suffering with some horrible disease for which there has been no real answer in the mainstream medical pharmacopeia, there always seems to appear, out of nowhere, legions of snake oil salesmen, medical magicians, and miracle products, all lining up to take your money, time, and precious energy. Pious-eyed and smiling, they will all claim they can transform your horrific malaise into wellness with the swipe of their magic wand and your credit card. And so began my shingles journey.

When I finally got over the shock that my doctor really didn't have much in the way of answers for my shingles (herpes zoster) outbreak, I suddenly realized, with no clue as to where to turn, it was every man for himself.

Aside from a single prescription drug that may or may not reduce the time of the shingles infection and may or may not prevent or shorten the life of resulting post-herpetic neuralgia (PHN), it is quite possible that your regular doctor can't help you – that is, unless you're willing to chance opioid, antiseizure, antidepressant, and palliative prescriptions that may bring their own subset of health problems. The single front-line prescription drug on offer is any one of a trio of _ciclovir solutions that turn out to be hit-or-miss. In my case, Valaciclovir and later Famciclovir did not help - at all. Initially, in my panicked clamor to find some sort of remedy for a painful shingles outbreak, I was one of those that had his wallet lightened by get-well-quick products and services that did not help. I was desperate. Shingles pain makes you crazy.

The purpose of my booklet is to inform so that interested readers do not waste their time chasing wrong answers and spending money on placebos that offer nothing but false hope. The intent is to provide, at the very least, tools to help navigate around the labyrinth of real and imagined help for this terrible disease, and, ideally, a protocol that will help relieve the symptoms and remediate the herpes zoster infection.

Shingles Relief! focuses on solutions for relief from the pain, burning and itching associated with the disease, and an in-depth look at remedies that promote rapid healing. It also focuses on what didn't work for me, and promising protocols that I didn't try, that might work well for some people. Detailed background material about the nature of the herpes zoster virus, and PHN is already abundantly available on the Internet, and I will not go over that material again in this volume.

The information in *Shingles Relief!* is based on my real life, first-hand experience, my interviews with doctors (alternative and allopathic, some of whom had shingles) and patients who were either suffering with the disease or who had toughed it out and gotten past it, a great deal of research, and my own endless experimentation with different modalities, successful and not so successful. There are no miracles in this booklet, only small, incremental victories in a battle that initially looked hopeless.

Although I did satisfy the course and grade requirements for application to medical school, my university degrees are not in medicine and I am not affiliated with any company that sells drugs, natural remedies or medical services. Any references to product names, companies, or practitioners in this booklet are for clarification purposes only. I do not profit from the sale of or from the promotion of any medical professional or any natural or medical product, drug or treatment regimen. For this reason, I do not endorse any of the latter. It is up to the reader to establish in his or her mind the credibility of any given product, service or protocol. This booklet recounts the author's personal experience with this disease and resulting conclusions. My hope is that, after reading *Shingles Relief!*, the reader will be in a much better position to find the best solution for a rapid and complete remission from a herpes zoster infection.

As I've mentioned, in order to not waste the reader's time, I try not to rehash here what is already readily available on the web. Many of you have picked up this booklet because you are looking for solutions and are probably not in the mood to be entertained by interesting trivia about shingles. Because of this, I have provided a number of web links in the appendix, and throughout the text, for those of you who are interested in doing further research into specific subjects of interest.

It is my wish that those of you who are suffering with this disease will find accelerated relief using one of the protocols talked about in this booklet. At the very least, I have attempted to provide a solid baseline and map from which to start an efficient and effective search to find real answers for shingles suffering.

Part 1 - Yikes Shingles!

It comes out of nowhere and most people don't even know what it is when they first get it. No one is spared. People over 60 experience it more, but anyone at nearly any age can fall victim. You can be a physical specimen or a walking disaster area, it doesn't matter.

There's a vaccine for it, but it's efficacy has been downgraded to somewhere between 18% to 51%, and the bad news is, the vaccine becomes less effective the older you get, providing the very group that needs it most with the least amount of protection. It gets scarier when you realize that mainstream medicine has precious little to offer shingles sufferers. When you first get it, they will offer you one of a trio of _ciclovir prescription drugs that may, or may not, shorten the term of the infection and may, or may not, provide you with protection from the dreaded postherpetic neuralgia (PHN) that can accompany this disease, lasting months after the disease itself has subsided.

Chapter 1
Scared Sailors and Sinking Ships

There is an old sailor's saying that goes something like this: "There is no finer bilge pump on a sinking ship than a scared sailor with a 5-gallon bucket in his hands."

I was that scared sailor. Shingles is horrific, especially when you get it in the face and eye or eyes. I desperately needed to find real answers to an excruciating disease that came out of nowhere and stopped my life cold in its tracks. I had ophthalmic shingles. I had it on the right side of my head and face and in my right eye. The epithelial layer of my cornea became frosted as a result of the disease, and my iris was infected and malfunctioning as a result. I was effectively blind in my right eye. The pain and extreme sensitivity on the right side of my head was excruciating and was persistent, 24/7, with no relief in sight.

My father always impressed upon us the importance of good health in life. "Health is your most important asset," he would say. The advice stuck. I have always tried to maintain good dietary habits, a regular exercise routine, and abstinence from drugs, alcohol and environments that were toxic. This shingles infection came out of nowhere. I was shocked.

Being a writer I now found myself instantly out of business, no longer able to even look at a computer or read a book for more than a few minutes because of the nerve damage around my eye. Even putting an ear plug in my right ear was an endurance test that had to be cut short after listening for just a short while.

I could not lie down. The pain would quadruple every time I tried to lay my head down. I had to try to sleep sitting upright, every single night for more than two and a half weeks. I was exhausted, weak, in extreme pain and finding nothing or anyone that could help.

At the beginning of the outbreak, I was nauseous, vomiting every half hour to 45 minutes or so. I was forced to adopt a strategy to keep from dehydrating - saltine crackers, ginger extract tablets and a water bottle nearby at all times. I didn't feel like eating - at all. I had to force myself to eat even though I had no appetite. My bowl movements were almost non-existent waiting sometimes nearly five days for something to happen. When I finally could, I downed an Epsom salt solution to force evacuation.

For the better part of two and a half weeks my only option was to sit up straight and nap - 24/7. I could not tolerate the usual diversions - no TV, computer, music through earphones (yikes!), smart phone or reading. The highlight of my day was to sleep. When I could. And later, to learn to meditate in an attempt to help transition the pain to subside, at least temporarily (more on this later). Any complications (sometimes referred to as cascading failures) during this period could have proven dangerous: harm, in any way, to the left eye, which was not injured, would have left me totally blind; a flu/other disease, or injury would have had serious consequences most likely requiring hospitalization or other supervised care. Shingles was a show stopper - a forced consciousness fast that I never asked for.

I was, indeed the scared sailor with the 5-gallon bucket in his hands and, as soon as I could, spent every possible moment looking for remediation options. I've learned a great deal during this journey and decided to share with other sufferers what I have learned.

Chapter 2
Off to Emergency!

I had no idea what was going on when I got shingles. As I said, during the night I had applied heat to a headachy area around my right eye and woke up with a feeling like I had hair growing around and into my eye, accompanied by a growing numbness, sensitivity and pain - and later, intense burning. There was a rash on the right side of my head extending around my right eye and covering the right side and down to the tip of my nose. I had no idea what it was.

At the time, I was ignorant about shingles. As a result I was concerned that this might be some sort of life threatening issue. I didn't suspect shingles.

I took myself to the local medical center emergency room. When I asked the triage nurse what she thought it was, she simply said, "you don't want to know . . . ." I thought for sure she was referring to some kind of physiological catastrophe, "well, this sucks, I guess I'm going to die now . . . ."

The attending physician was an ophthalmologist. He told me that it was a herpes zoster infection and that the eye was involved. He prescribed Valacyclovir which is an 'antiviral' drug designed to treat herpes infections. An appointment was scheduled with another ophthalmologist.

Before I left, the nurse held out an 800mg Ibuprofen tablet for me to take - it looked like a buffalo pill - "take one of these, you'll feel better." I was hesitant, because this was the first time I had ever taken an over the counter pain medication. I took it anyway, like the scared sailor that I was.

Despite its extra strength size, the ibuprofen didn't seem to do anything to cause any of the discomfort to subside. And since there is a package warning about overdoses of Ibuprofen occurring after 3200 mg in a 24 hour period, I decided that I would quickly exceed the maximum dosage if I had any hope of experiencing some kind of relief from this medication. This same scenario played out again later on, as you will see, when the pain became even worse, this time attempting to get some relief with over-the-counter extra strength Tylenol. (See *What Didn't Work*)

An eye drug called erythromycin was also initially prescribed. This turned out to be an antibacterial drug, most commonly used for acne outbreaks.

Right after the emergency visit I went to the pharmacy and got the Valacyclovir and Erthromycin prescriptions. I went to the drinking fountain and I took a Valacyclovir immediately. The one gram dose was to be taken three times a day. After just one day on this drug I was experiencing side effects. and while the drowsiness, mood changes, increased thirst, loss of appetite, nausea and vomiting may have been part and parcel of the disease itself, the drug seemed to noticeably exacerbate these issues.

At the appointment with the ophthalmologist I told him about the problem with Valacyclovir and asked to try Famciclovir, a more recent iteration of the _ciclovir 'antiviral' trio of drugs. This was a 500mg 4x a day dosage that was well tolerated - I was easily able to get through the entire course with no noticeable side effects.

Strictly speaking, the _ciclovir family of 'antiviral' drugs are not truly antiviral. The 'anti' in antibacterial, antiviral, and antifungal usually implies that the drug kills the disease agent. The various _ciclovir drugs do not kill anything. What they are supposed to do is slow the growth and spread of the herpes virus in the body. They do *not* cure or kill herpes viruses. Also, there is a claim made for these drugs that they will reduce the possibility of the patient experiencing post-herpetic neuralgia (PHN) after the shingle infection subsides. You don't want to know what this is . . . but I'll tell you anyway. PHN is the residue pain you are left with after the shingles infection subsides. A shingles infection will damage nerves. That damage can be severe enough to where you may never recover from it.

The Valaciclovir and Famciclovir prescription drugs that I took did not prevent PHN, in my case. And yes, I followed doctor's instructions exactly and the drug was taken in a timely fashion. Not only did the drug not eliminate the possibility of PHN, in my case, there is some doubt as to whether the drug actually did anything at all.

The erythromycin prescription was troublesome to me. I spoke to the ophthalmologist about this and he confirmed that it was an antibacterial drug. The reason for the prescription was to protect the eye from possible bacterial contamination. My gut feeling was to wait before applying this - a call that turned out to be accurate.

After carefully analyzing the damage to the eye, on this very first visit, the ophthalmologist prescribed a 1% prednisolone eye drop solution to be applied four times daily. Prednisolone is a steroid drug, which, if misused, can cause damage to the cornea, among other things. At 1% solution I felt it was worth trying, as the eye problem was acute and there was a great deal of anxiety at the time about regaining my eyesight. Following the prescription order, I put 1 drop in my eye 4 times a day. Whether this drug actually helped or not, is difficult to say. The eye has impressive regenerative/recuperative abilities on its own, and I didn't want to interfere with this natural process either. But, again, I was the scared sailor with the 5-gallon bucket in his hands, so I was going to go with whatever program was presented during this initial stage of illness.

Successive visits to the ophthalmologist's office yielded little in the way of real help, but mostly just analysis designed to monitor the progress of the healing. It became clearer, after several weeks of visits to doctors, that there really is no solution available from mainstream medicine, either for the remediation of the disease or its symptoms. None that would make any sense. When this finally hit me, there was a brief wave of panic - like when you realize that, despite all efforts, the scared sailor may not be able to bail fast enough to save his sinking ship.

Chapter 3
Why me???

Onset

I could not understand why I became a victim of this hideous disease. I really go out of my way to take good care of myself, and always have. I eat healthy and I'm an active outdoors person who gets regular exercise, fresh air and sunshine. I've never abused drugs or alcohol and I've never smoked. I guess I'm pretty boring, actually. So, do boring people get shingles?

After I got down off my pity potty and started doing some research I found out why people get this disease. There seems to be a very definite precursor pattern to a Shingles outbreak - and my situation seemed a classic example. Since then, I have come up with a list of what I experienced to be the precursors for the infection.

1. You've had chickenpox in the past.

2. You are experiencing, and doing nothing about persistent stress in your life.

3. Your body's lysine levels are low. Foods with high arginine/lysine ratios may help to maintain low levels of lysine which may create an environment for herpes (high

levels of arginine may lower lysine levels in the body; high levels of arginine has been implicated in the proliferation of the herpes virus). You are consistently eating foods with a high arginine ratio (see *Being Proactive*)

4. You are ignoring persistent low grade neuralgic-type pain or highly unusual sensations in areas where shingles is known to appear on the body (head, face, torso) and . . .

5. The area in question (above) is subject to exposure of persistent warming or heat.

I'll explain from the perspective of my case.

Chickenpox

As a child, I remember having chickenpox. At the time, it was common. It seemed like everyone had it. You get over it. You forget it. That is, until you get shingles.

Stress

The several months before my outbreak, I was experiencing constant, low grade stress to make deadlines. This was by no means traumatic stress, just the constant goading of just-under-the-radar stress to get work done. Because of it, I seemed to be definitely more edgy and measurably less patient than normal. As an aside, every one of the shingles sufferers that I talked to said that they felt stress played a role in precipitating the outbreak.

Persistent pain

For months, I had a persistent pain over, and just to the side of my right eye which I attributed to using plain magnifier-type reading glasses rather than prescription computer glasses. My right eye lagged in vision acuity versus my left eye. I kept promising to get prescription glasses, but I didn't. The pain was not acute, but was a mild to moderate distraction that often caused me to take breaks away from my work on the computer in order to give this pain a chance to subside a bit.

Lysine/arginine ratio

One of my favorite foods is blueberries. I mean, really favorite. Costco sells three-pound bags of frozen organic blueberries at a reasonable price, and I would buy them and devour the contents of three or more bags per month, ofttimes just making a meal out of them. I did this for several months. What I didn't know (and didn't care about at the time) was that blueberries are very similar to nuts and seeds in their lysine /arginine ratio, heavily favoring arginine. Excessive arginine has been implicated in fostering an environment receptive to herpes outbreaks. While I get plenty of lysine in my regular diet, this huge intake of an arginine weighted food very likely may have helped to tip the balance, helping, in part, to support a shingles outbreak. (see the *appendix* section of the booklet for links to websites for in-depth discussions about the lysine/arginine ratio as it relates to herpes zoster/shingles)

Heat as a precursor to imminent outbreak

Shingles Relief!

As I said, before the outbreak, I was bothered by the persistent pain over, and to the side of, my right eye. Long story short, in one of my attempts to get the pain to subside I applied heat to the area. What I didn't know then was that the kind of zoster outbreak that I experienced is encouraged by persistent warmth and heat. It was precisely when I applied heat that the shingles outbreak occurred - with a vengeance. The timing was perfect: pain in that area for months, but certainly no sign of anything resembling shingles; the very first application of heat resulted in an outbreak. There was such a precise correlation that the application of the heat seemed to be an undeniable piece of this initial outbreak puzzle, in my mind (see *Being Proactive*, the section at the bottom of the chapter).

Chapter 4
Same Disease, Different Experiences

One of the reasons why it is so difficult to treat any disease is because of the way in which each individual manifests that disease and responds to treatment. Clinical trials, the standard in today's scientific approach to medical research, are often stymied by the reality of psychological and physiological idiosyncrasies, one person to the next, making drugs and protocols that appeared effective during trials, to be highly unreliable among some in the general population.

A shingles outbreak on the chest, back or buttocks may have very different implications than an outbreak across the eye, face, or head. For some sufferers, heat, for example, may exacerbate the terrible symptoms, while, for others, cold will be a problem. Duration of infection, chances of PHN after the infection, and sensitivities to the disease will vary by individual and location of infection. Regardless of variability, however, there are baseline commonalities. This book focuses on these, allowing for the same healing modalities to address different iterations of the disease.

Responses to therapy will vary as well. While some may get benefit from one of the _ciclovir prescription drugs, others will experience no benefit whatsoever. The latter is what I experienced. While high-dose B12 regimens work very well for some, as in my case, homeopathic cocktails may work better for others. Again, there is a baseline of shared shingles traits that are core target factors when looking for relief.

I will address those in upcoming chapters as I talk about which protocols, substances, regimens and treatments worked, which might have worked, and which didn't work for me.

Chapter 5
Finding the Right Doctor

B efore I begin the section on what worked and what didn't, I want to impress upon the reader how important it is to find the right doctor to work with at the very beginning of the outbreak of shingles. This could save valuable time and money, and reduce healing time and suffering considerably. I can't emphasize this enough.

When I got sick with shingles, my first instinct, and probably yours, was that I should go to my regular doctor immediately (regular doctor meaning mainstream, allopathic, medical doctor). While this is a good idea, in the end it turned out not to be very useful to me. As I have said elsewhere, mainstream medicine really does not have much of an answer for a shingles infection, but because many of us don't know where else to turn – or because that's all our insurance will cover – we keep going back in the hopes they will take pity and dig deep into their little black medicine bag and pull out something miraculous. But they won't. And the faster you move on and find competent alternative help, the quicker you will be on your way to healing.

One of my big wish list items while I was sick was to be able to find a doctor who would be willing to work with me in trying a broader spectrum of natural and allopathic remedies and protocols. For example, it would have been wonderful to have found a doctor who was knowledgeable about injectable high-dose B12 and high-dose C treatments, or who was willing to administer a full capsicum treatment protocol (in office). Initially, I had little luck where I live. While there are some good naturopathic doctors in my area, the prohibitive cost of trying different ones out to see which one was familiar with successful shingles and PHN remediation protocols was a real disincentive.

In my case, I had already been bilked of my time, money and energy. through my own ignorance, by pharmaceutical, medical, and natural remedies that were nothing more than wishful thinking, and was becoming very skeptical about ever finding an honest third-party solution. I learned the hard way that it is worth the time and effort from the very outset of the disease to look for and then work with a credible practitioner who is familiar with a wide range of natural and allopathic remedies. I know this is starting to sound like a broken record but, mainstream medicine does not really have an answer for shingles, so it is quite possible that your regular doctor will not be able to help you. One possible exception would be the medical doctor who has a degree in Integrative Medicine, or one who also holds a degree in naturopathy.

I later learned from a local naturopath that, for example, high dosages of B12 were very beneficial. This was the turning point in my suffering with this disease, and the benefits from this one tip proved invaluable. From my research, intravenous injections of B12 seems to have gotten the nod most often. But, because I couldn't find a doctor who did this, I ended up taking high dosages of B12 sublingually, which turned out to work well enough (see *What Worked*). Doctors who have taken the time to educate themselves in the broader spectrum of solutions can often get you prescription grade products that would truly help - products that mainstream allopathic physicians might not know about.

As I eluded to above, going off the mainstream medical beaten path will probably cost you out-of-pocket. Sadly, our medical system is so locked into prescription pharmaceutical protocols, that insurance companies refuse to pay for treatments or professional services that are unwilling to go down this road. Even FDA approved scenar devices (see *What Might Work)* in the hands of trained medical doctors are not approved for payment by insurers.

All is not lost, there are still ways to make alternative treatment doable, despite the cost. This might be one area where friends and family could help out, or the practitioner may be willing to spread the cost out over time, in payments. Family and friends who provide assistance in helping to find a competent practitioner, and temporarily fund a visit, at least in part, would be making an amazing gift to a shingles sufferer.

One word of caution. Because of the hordes of charlatans that prey on those desperate for a solution to this illness, it is very important to vet your choice of doctors carefully. The Internet makes this a little easier, but talk to as many people as possible about your choice of doctors before committing. During your vetting process, talk to the doctor and ask specific questions about their experience with shingles treatment. If he or she doesn't seem to have the time to satisfactorily answer your questions, move on to the next one.

So, who is the right doctor?
Firstly, the right doctor fully understands the nature of the disease, and its implications, and can competently direct a patient to seek treatment that is appropriate inside and *outside* of mainstream medicine.

Good candidates are osteopathic and naturopathic doctors, and MDs who practice Integrative medicine. As a side note, there are clinics that are starting to pop up around the country that specialize in high-dose natural IV drips (like high-dose B12).

The right doctor:

1. Recognizes and is knowledgeable about alternative and mainstream shingles remediation and is prepared to administer and monitor protocols like, for example, intravenous injections of B12 and C, and other natural, non-prescription 'cocktails,' as determined.

2. Is knowledgeable about pain relief approaches like, for example, scenar and FSM microcurrent treatments and, if appropriate, can administer them or be able to recommend a physician who can do this effectively and efficiently.

3. Is knowledgeable about homeopathic and ayurvedic healing modalities as they apply to shingles.

4. Knows how to effectively manage symptoms without prescription opioids, steroids, or other dangerous drugs and can recommend a specific safe and effective protocol that has worked well for other shingles sufferers.

5. Makes the *time* to work collaboratively with his or her patients to find safe, efficient, effective solutions.

A quick way to vet doctors would be to tell them about the alternative protocols that you had in mind. Mainstream doctors like to discredit alternative remedies, or natural-based protocols, as 'Internet cures.' If the doctor you are considering refers to any of the components of the protocol listed in *What Worked,* in this book, as an "internet cure," quietly move on. That's all you need to know to disqualify that doctor. Too many mainstream doctors only vouch for protocols which require prescription pharmaceuticals. As I've already mentioned, the prescription drugs on offer for shingles are nothing more than snake oil for some, as in my case, while they might be useful for others. In my case, not only was there no benefit to the prescribed _ciclovirs, I suffered side effects when taking Valacyclovir.

The alternative components of the protocol listed in *What Worked* in this book all have mainstream scientific backing. Some are backed by double blind studies, others in vitro studies, and others, mainstream scientific research. So the doctor who calls them "Internet cures" chooses to be ignorant of the science behind this approach. Even the core concept behind the mind/body routine suggested in *What Worked* is backed by convincing double blind studies conducted by Harvard and Cambridge medical schools.

(Web search: The Power of the Placebo, studies by Harvard and Cambridge Universities; link: http://www.dailymotion.com/video/x1z4iyq_e07-the-power-of-the-placebo_tv).

As an aside, less convincing are the scientific studies conducted by pharmaceutical companies to prove the efficacy and safety of the prescription drugs that they would like to market to the public. This comment by Dr. Marcia Angell, Harvard medical school professor and editor for the New England Journal of Medicine, for some twenty years, sums it up:

"It is simply no longer possible to believe much of the clinical research that is published, or to rely on the judgment of trusted physicians or authoritative medical guidelines. I take no pleasure in this conclusion, which I reached slowly and reluctantly over my two decades as an editor of The New England Journal of Medicine."

Because shingles outbreaks are common, there is a good chance that there is a practitioner near you that can help. The right practitioner can help with solutions to abbreviate the length and damaging effects of this disease.

Chapter 6
Understanding Alternative Remedies for Shingles

Because mainstream medicine has little on offer for shingles patients, alternative remedies, supplements and medications become the focus of many sufferer's searches. Unfortunately, this area of healthcare is unregulated and, in some cases, poorly understood, and the snake oil salesmen are many who would take your money for products that may offer nothing in exchange. Below is a list of credible natural products that should be a part of a larger protocol that is meant to bring about shingles relief. The list was a product of much research, interviews with patients and doctors, and considerable personal experimentation.

L-lysine: Anyone doing research on shingles remediation will almost immediately run into a discussion about lysine and its relationship to a herpes infection. While there still hasn't been a lot of medical research on this subject, the avalanche of testimonials avowing to lysine's role in shingles remediation is impressive. There has also been some interesting work at the University of Maryland on this subject (http://umm.edu/health/medical/altmed/supplement/lysine).

Lysine is not naturally produced in the body and must be provided by dietary choices. In my own case, there is certainly compelling evidence to suggest that a lysine deficit may have played a role in creating an environment for a zoster outbreak. I had been eating huge quantities of organic blueberries for several months before my shingles outbreak, sometimes just substituting the blueberries for a normal meal. Blueberries are extremely high in arginine, an amino acid that is known to deplete lysine levels and encourage herpes replication in the body.

This does not mean that arginine is an undesirable substance. Quite the contrary. Arginine, naturally produced in the body, is, among other things, implicated in the repair of peripheral neuropathy, a form of PHN, a condition that some shingles sufferers experience after their zoster infection has subsided. Lysine and arginine exist in a balanced relationship and, especially in the post infection, PHN stages, arginine is important.

Monolaurin: found in coconut milk and breast milk, monolaurin is used specifically to fight viral infections, including the common cold and shingles. The purest form of monolaurin is supposedly found in a product called Lauricidin, but it is not clear if other versions of this non-prescription drug/supplement are less potent.

There have been a number of studies verifying the efficacy of monolaurin against viral infections making this a good choice in the arsenal of an effective shingles relief protocol.

For a more in depth discussion about monolaurin and shingles see: http://www.advancedhealing.com/antiviral-antibacterial-actions-of-monolaurin-and-lauric-acid/

Moducare: contains sterols and sterolins which have been shown to bolster immune system health. Your single greatest asset in the fight against shingles, or any disease, is the health of your immune system. If your immune system were perfectly healthy, then a zoster infection would most likely subside relatively quickly, or, perhaps, never have appeared in the first place. Immune system boosters have a place in a comprehensive shingles remediation protocol.

Melissa Officinalis, or **Lemon Balm:** Discovering this well-known herb when searching for herpes zoster remedies is almost unavoidable. Lemon balm topical ointment has been effective in accelerating the healing of a shingles infection. Less convincing for shingles is the tea and capsule forms, which have better reputations as sedatives and mood enhancers.

Vitamin C: It seems Linus Pauling's successes with vitamin C therapies have somehow given license to vitamin C being a kind of cure-all for everything. While I'm sure vitamin C is absolutely essential for various healthy physiological processes, high-dose vitamin C therapy, by itself, may not be enough to bring relief from shingles. However, because vitamin C is not produced naturally in the body, and because it supports good health in so many basic cellular functions, and because it purportedly has antiviral properties, a high-dose vitamin C regimen is a credible component in a shingles and PHN remediation regimen. I didn't try injectable C mainly because I couldn't find a practitioner that would do this, so I took it in a high dose, buffered, capsule form.

Vitamin B12: Injectable versions of B12 protocols would be more effective than capsule intake. However, there are single-stage high dose B12 products that are assimilated quickly and tolerated quite well that may be a very acceptable substitute (single-stage examples: Natural Factors methylcobalamin B12, 5,000mcg chewable or sublingual tablets; Costco's Kirkland brand methylcobalamin B12, 5,000mcg chewable or sublingual tablets, the latter being considerably less expensive). In my own case, I responded extremely well to this protocol, which I will discuss further in the chapter on *What Worked*. Generally, high dosages of B12 are safe for extended periods, for most people. One caveat, if you are pregnant or have a medical condition besides shingles, see comments about B12 side effects here: Web search: side effects of high-dose vitamin B12;

link: http://www.webmd.com/vitamins-supplements/ingredientmono-926-vitamin%20b12.aspx?activeingredientid=926.

Vitamin B6: another of the B vitamins that directly enhances nerve health and may be very beneficial in helping to relieve and remediate nerve damage caused by shingles and PHN.

The caveat about B6 is that, in high doses, unlike B12, side effects can occur that can be quite dangerous. This is one of those instances where taking higher doses of a vitamin needs careful planning. Super high doses probably should be done under the supervision of a doctor. In any event, monitor dosages carefully.

B-complex vitamins: taken in combination with B6 and B12, as noted above, a good quality B-complex supplement can be part of a successful shingles protocol. The B vitamins, in general, and B6 and B12 in particular, help to restore and maintain some nervous system components. The shingles virus wreaks havoc in the neural pathways that it infects, often leaving nerve damage that sometimes can last a lifetime. Getting started on a good B-complex regimen along with high dose B6 and B12 supplements, will, from my own experience, go a long way in helping to remediate this nerve damage. Again, note the dosage restrictions applied to B6.

Vitamin E (mixed natural tocopherols may be best): At least one study has shown the potential effectiveness of higher dose vitamin E treatment, particularly for the pain associated with a shingles infection and postherpetic neuralgia (important note: if taking aspirin or other blood thinner, discuss your plan to take higher dosages of vitamin E with a doctor first)

Capsicum (Capsaicin): In my experience, capsicum capsules were not helpful in giving me relief from my shingles pain. I may not have given them a fair trial, though, because later I did find that eating jalapeno peppers helped quite a bit! Capsicum Ointment treatments might be more effective (Zostrix or Capzasin-P), but I deliberately did not try these because of my extreme sensitivity to heat of any kind. Localized capsicum treatments, done in a doctor's office with prescription grade capsicum, may be effective for long-term pain relief, especially where PHN is the primary culprit. Ask your practitioner if he or she is familiar with this treatment.

Tumeric (Curcuma) for pain relief; I tried Zyflamend which contains, among other herbs, tumeric. Zyflamend appears to be an excellent quality product, but it wasn't able to provide even the slightest relief for my zoster pain or discomfort. I was left doubting whether turmeric, even ingested in its pure form, would have any effect on shingles-related pain. However, tumeric, made into a paste and applied topically, may be useful in helping particularly PHN pain to subside. I did not try this because the very idea of putting something warm on the affected area was not an option. Other sufferers may not have a problem with this option.

Acupuncture: Although I was not in a position to try acupuncture (and this turned out to be a significant omission in my original attempt to treat my shingles infection) acupuncture combined with moxibustion has been found in clinical trials to be more effective than the neuro-pharaceutical Gabapentin (neurontin) in treating shingles.

Shingles Relief!

(http://www.healthcmi.com/Acupuncture-Continuing-Education-News/1314-acupuncture-beats-drugs-for-shingles-nerve-pain)

There is voluminous material about this subject on the web and I will not rehash that here. Suffice it to say that acupuncture can play a significant role in accelerating shingles relief. Again, finding the right doctor, or doctors, is crucial to your speedy recovery from a shingles infection. In this case you may need to find a knowledgeable naturopathic doctor or eastern medicine doctor and an acupuncture doctor. Well worth the effort, especially when you consider the considerable benefits. The chances of a dreaded PHN aftermath, as a result of a shingles infection, decreases dramatically in cases where the original shingles infection is dealt with quickly and effectively. In other words, the faster you get shingles under control, the less likely it is that you will experience postherpetic neuralgia.

Homeopathic Remedies: the use of homeopathic remedies for shingles has been successful in the hands of trained homeopathic practitioners. I was unable to find a qualified homeopathic practitioner and so did not have a chance to try this. When looking for the right doctor, ask if he or she is familiar with homeopathic remedies for shingles. If they are not, chances are they may not be the right person to see about a zoster infection, as most naturopathic practitioners are well acquainted with the homeopathic pharmacopeia . During my interviews with zoster veterans, I found at least one person who experienced convincing success with a homeopathic remedy administered by a practitioner. The following link will provide more information about homeopathic remedies for shingles: Web search: homeopathy for shingles; link: http://www.naturalnews.com/039071_shingles_homeopathic _remedies_pain_relief.html

Healing sessions (meditative breath and guided imagery sessions to enhance natural healing): If the body did not know how to heal itself, there wouldn't be a single one of us left on the planet. We would have long ago perished. Doctors, especially surgeons, seem to almost dismiss this out of hand. In fact, there couldn't exist even the most minor surgical procedure without the self healing that occurs naturally in every living thing. Mind/body interaction with regards to physiology has been well known to the mainstream medical community. With the advent of Psychoneuroimmunology (PNI), a relatively new discipline within allopathic medicine, scientists are now trying to understand this phenomenon.

Essentially, I realized that the healing that I was looking for was going to take place inside of me, and not solely as a result of some third party intervention. I know that the body is perfectly equipped to take care of itself and that I seemed to be getting in the way of this process more than I probably should have. There is no instant gratification in this method – no instant fix – but using the technique patiently, along with other suggested protocols in this booklet, helped bring about results, in my case. See *What Worked - The Mind Body Connection*.

Water Treatments: I discovered the benefits of exposure to light-pressure tap water sessions quite by accident when I was desperately looking for some way to take the edge off the hideous 24/7 pain, itching, and burning that comes with every zoster infection. None of the over the counter medications helped, and my regular doctor had no answers. The discomfort was driving me mad. (See the section on *What Worked - Water Water Everywhere*). At one point, a naturopath eluded to the benefits of running water over the area when she suggested spraying iWater (ionized water) on my shingles outbreak 10x a day. I'm not convinced about the efficacy ionized water, but the light-pressure tap water idea that I had already stumbled upon was working well, so I didn't see a need to change what I was doing.

Part 2 - What Worked and What Didn't

Some of you have probably skipped right to this section of the booklet. I certainly don't blame you. During my infection, all I was looking for was relief!

In this section I'm not going to review information you could just as easily get off the web, so I will give you an overview, from my experience, about what I actually found with each of these touted 'remedies' or 'important contributors' to shingles remediation and/or management. If the reader wants to do more research on specific topics, I have provided links in the appendix section of this booklet.

Chapter 7
What Didn't Work

Prescription Drugs and Remedies

The following mainstream, first line, prescription drugs did not work for me:

Valaciclovir: during the visit to the emergency room, the doctor prescribed 1,000mg dosages of this drug, 3x a day. In a very short time, I was experiencing side effects and switched to Famciclovir in dosages of 500mg , 4x a day.

Famciclovir: I took this drug as directed. It should also be noted that I took these _ciclovir drugs in a timely fashion, well within 72 hours of the shingles outbreak. Calling these drugs antiviral is a bit of a stretch. Antibacterial, antifungal, or 'anti' anything refers to the fact that the drug kills off the disease agent, in this case, the viruses. In actual fact, the _ciclovirs kill off nothing, and do not cure shingles, or any herpes virus, but, instead, create an environment, theoretically, where the virus cannot continue to infect or spread, thus, supposedly shortening the life of the infection. In actual fact, in my case, the drug did not shorten the life cycle of the infection (I had the infection itself for just over two and a half weeks, with absolutely no sign of relief or remission before starting on the protocol listed in *What Worked*). Further, none of the prescription drugs protected me against resulting PHN, which lasted for two months after the infection abated.

Interesting side note, the doctor who was treating me said that if the PHN continued over a long period of time, neurologists might recommend opioids, a potentially dangerous class of drugs, for pain remediation.

 Prescribed, too, was prednisolone eye drop solution: This prescription eye medicine was intended to help my right eye recover from the damage caused by the shingles intrusion. This drug may have been helpful, but I have no way of being sure. On two occasions ophthalmologists have reminded me that the eye is very resilient and has great recuperative capabilities, without the help of medications. Natural remission may have been more a factor in my eye healing than anything to do with the prednisolone. As I said, I have no way of knowing for sure.

A word about the shingles vaccine

When Merck first released its Zostavax (shingles vaccine), the expectation was that the drug would be at least 70% - 90% effective in preventing a zoster outbreak. Unfortunately, since that time, the latest research indicates that the $200-per-jab vaccine may only be anywhere from 18% to 51% effective, depending on age group (effectiveness declining with age). There are a number of other unsettling questions about the vaccine that have arisen, as well, but I won't rehash that here.

In the appendix section, I have provided links to some websites that discuss this information in depth for those who are interested. One thing for sure, if there is no history of a chickenpox outbreak during childhood, chances are there is little or no chance of a shingles outbreak later on in life. I would not even consider a Zostavax vaccine if there were no history of chickenpox.

Natural Substances (herbal and vitamin supplements, oils, creams, capsules)

First of all, none of the natural substances that I tried were, by themselves, helpful in bringing me relief. (see Understanding the Natural Pharmacopeia as Remedies for Shingles). However, as part of a complete, multi-faceted protocol, several of the natural substances and therapies were, indeed valuable. I will discuss in more detail in *What Worked*, what these substances are, what protocols they are used in, and how they worked for me. You may be surprised at some of what I found that worked well.

Aloe Vera. Surprisingly, I did not find aloe vera cream to be helpful. Aloe, in other contexts, has been a life saver for me. I buy aloe in creams and in one gallon juice containers. I use it often, and I tried using the light cream on my shingles rash. I was quite confident that there would be results. But there weren't, and after a brief period of time, I gave up on it. I know that you will read, during your web searches, about how well aloe works on shingles rashes. I had no such luck with it and did not continue to incorporate it into my regimen.

However, having said that, I did not try spraying aloe juice from a spray bottle onto the infected area, just as I had done with regular water. The aloe juice that I am referring to is the light viscosity, water-like juice that you can buy in gallons for around $10. This might, indeed, have some merit and would be worth trying (see *What Might Work*)

Over the Counter Medications (OTC)

Generally, over the counter medications are lightweights when it comes to this infection. Here's a rundown of what I tried:

Ibuprofen (for pain relief): I took the extra strength version (800mg) of this OTC med and it was useless. First of all, it didn't come close to taking the edge off the terrible pain. Second of all, if it had been able to take the edge off, I would have had to have taken so much of it that I would have put myself at severe risk of some of the more serious side effects of this drug. How serious? Heart attack, stroke, bleeding intestines, bleeding stomach, etc. For the curious, have a look at this well-known website: https://www.drugs.com/ibuprofen.html

Motrin IB (for pain relief): the main ingredient in this OTC med is ibuprofen. See above. I tried Motrin for a short time, on the advice of a neighbor, and, of course, had the same experience as when I took ibuprofen, above.

Tylenol (for pain relief): This acetaminophen OTC med was a little useful in taking some of the edge off the pain. However, I was having to take 1,000mg every three hours which meant that I could not get anywhere near around-the-clock relief. I could, at most, take this med for nine hours worth of relief before I would start to get into the overdose range. The other 15 hours, I was out of luck. Overdosing on Tylenol is the leading cause of liver failure in the United States today. You don't want to take more than 4,000mg of this OTC drug in any 24 our period.

Lidocaine patches (topical pain relief): I had little luck with these. There was some small relief for a very short period of time. I think you would need to reapply patches quite often. This would be impractical at the hairline, for example, where the patch would not be able to lie against the skin.

Lidocaine cream (topical pain relief): again, minimal relief. If you've got a zoster infection on your head, face and/or around your eyes, this could be very risky business. Getting even the slightest amount of Lidocaine cream in your eye during a shingles infection would be very painful.

Tri Derma Pain Relief Cream: the label on this OTC topical cream states that this is specifically for shingles pain (among other causes). I used this and found that the cream was nice and light and somewhat effective in taking the edge off the pain and burning. I have other TriDerma products, and like them. But, the relief from this product was too short-lived to be really practical. After a day or so, I abandoned this and continued with another method that turned out to be very effective (I will talk more about this in the chapter on *What Worked*).

Capsicum based creams (topical pain relief): I did not try capsicum creams. I suspect that the results, at least in my case, would have been much the same as with Lidocaine cream. In my case, heat around my infection was absolutely not welcome and the thought of the heat from capsicum scared me.

Having said this, capsicum creams and patches applied topically to an area affected by PHN has been successful for some people in helping to relieve pain. Capsicum is by no means a cure for PHN pain, but can help manage it. Again, I didn't try this, but there is a great deal of testimony to capsicum's success for some sufferers. See: http://www.ncbi.nlm.nih.gov/pmc/articles/PMC3169333/

Over the Counter Eye Medications

Because my eye was implicated in my shingles infection, I became the de facto guinea pig for OTC eye drops testing when the eye started showing signs of recovery. Here's what I found.

Bausch and Lomb Soothe Lubricant Eye Drops: This worked fairly well, lubricating and rehydrating the eye, but was only a short-term fix. The single-dispenser applicators are a pain in the neck and, to me, just seemed gimmicky.

Tears Naturale II Lubricating Eye Drops: this did not work well for me. I stopped using this OTC eye drop.

Systane Ultra Lubricant Eye Drops: these worked well for me, lubricating and rehydrating the eye while having the longest lasting effect. This turned out to be a keeper.

Generally speaking, I didn't have much luck with the OTC stuff. In my desperation for relief, I spent quite a bit of money on these medications. In hind sight, I'd skip them entirely and spend my time and money on better-documented protocols specific to shingles (for some ideas, see *What Worked*).

Scenar (Microcurrent) Treatment Using a TENs Unit

Because of the incredible discomfort and pain that I was suffering, I spent more money than I could afford on so-called scenar treatments. My medical insurance did not cover this option. The scenar method was invented in Russia and further developed by doctors here in the U.S. This therapy uses a device called a Tennant Biomodulator which relies on biofeedback from the damaged nerve to serve as a basis for electro stimulation. It was represented to me as a sure way to relieve a fair amount, at least, of the neural pain discomfort caused by the zoster virus. Long story short, aside from very brief periods of relief, the treatments did not help me. The doctor, who was an MD, got my money and I got some very painful trips to the doctor's office in exchange, and that was about it.

This brought up an interesting question. Why is it that doctors get paid anyway, even when they provide absolutely nothing of value for the patient - or worse, kill or injure the patient as we see in so many iatrogenic incidences every year? Certainly, if the medical community was disallowed payment for patient failures, I think advancements in medical treatment would skyrocket. Those doctors who say they'd walk away from medicine if this came about would be doing us all a favor, because they would make room for a new generation of doctors that would not only eagerly embrace a much broader base of remediation possibilities, but would also embrace proactive medicine, as advocates of healthy lifestyles.

Despite my experience with scenar, my own feeling was that this technique might have worked (see *What Might Work*) had the doctor been willing to apply the treatment twice daily for two full weeks or until the pain subsided. As it was, he kept scheduling me for appointments that were a week or more apart. In this scenario, there could be no cumulative effect, as the pain would quickly reassert itself resulting in no gains.

There is, however, encouraging news about other kinds of microcurrent treatments. There is a type of microcurrent treatment that is available by credible clinics and practitioners that has enjoyed considerable success treating pain associated with shingles and resulting PHN. This type of treatment is referred to as Frequency-Specific Microcurrent treatment (or FSM) and is available at some well known facilities like, for example the Cleveland Clinic. (for more information about this method: http://my.clevelandclinic.org/health/treatments_and_proced ures/hic-frequency-specific-microcurrent)

EFT/Tapping

EFT/Tapping (search key words EFT/Tapping on YouTube) utilizes acupressure points and guided imagery to help optimize health and to aid in the healing process. I am already somewhat familiar with the benefits of acupressure and guided imagery, so I tried EFT/tapping for a while to see how it would work. What I found was that it provided some relief, mainly, I think, because it helped distract my focus away from the pain and burning for a short while. In fact, distraction (I.e., momentarily removing your focus from the suffering) may be a useful temporary relief from the pain, burning and itching associated with a shingles outbreak - but it doesn't appear to me that it will cause the basis for the symptoms to actually subside.

Chapter 8
What Might Work

As I said, out of pure desperation I did a great deal of research on which credible remedies, substances, protocols and treatments were available to shingles sufferers. I ran across some interesting information about this subject, which may be worthwhile to some sufferers. I tried some of these, and some I didn't (indicated below). I'd like to share these with you here. Most of you will have already looked at the *What Worked* chapter. I've included this section to help broaden your basis for potential options.

Propolis

The propolis claim for zoster remediation is a slippery slope, in my opinion, because the labels on some propolis containers do not indicate product origin or much about how it was manufactured. There is a claim that the Propolis made from Manuka honey hives (only found in New Zealand), is the only truly effective propolis. Apparently, just picking up any old jar of propolis (pricey from any manufacturer) and applying the contents, may not even come close to solving shingles or PHN problems. I tried a 'propolis' from my local health food store. Small jar, giant letters PROPOLIS on the front. Very pricey. No sign of ingredient origin on the label. My understanding is that the actual bee hive comb itself forms the basis for the propolis end product. But some manufacturers sell propolis extract that may not necessarily be from honey comb. So, it's not clear, exactly, which propolis might be effective in treating shingles. Long story short, putting propolis from the jar to my herpes lesions did nothing but exacerbate the itchiness and pain, I think mainly because the substance acted as an insulating layer making the area feel warm, something that was very uncomfortable in my case. I stopped using it after just two applications.

As if to confuse things more, there was a clinical trial done on one specific type of 3% propolis-based product. The clinical trial demonstrated that patients did get relief from this particular product. The thing to remember about clinical trials is that they use very specific versions of a substance, sometimes not easily available on the market. While I have been able to find versions of this product on the web, for example, Herstat, I haven't seen it anywhere in the U.S. and couldn't get my hands on a package.

For more details about the tested efficacy of various drugs and natural substances for shingles see this University of Maryland web link: http://umm.edu/health/medical/altmed/condition/herpes-simplex-virus

Here is a website that features a useful in-depth discussion about various natural remedies for shingles and herpes,

including clinical studies information:
http://www.lifeextensionvitamins.com/heandshpa2.html

Aloe

I did not have much luck with aloe creams topically applied to my herpes rash. However, I did not try spraying or misting my infection with the 99.8% pure aloe juice that you can purchase in gallon containers at quite reasonable prices from places like Wal-Mart. Aloe in this latter form does not leave an unpleasant smell or residue and, with a viscosity like water, can be absorbed by the skin. As I said, I didn't try this, but it seems like a worthwhile experiment given the cost and convenience.

Apple Cider Vinegar

I did not try this, but have read several reports of people using this to dry out and help clear up shingles lesions. Apple cider vinegar is inexpensive and can be applied easily to the infected area.

Microcurrent Treatments: Scenar and FSM

I revisit microcurrent therapies here because they show promise in helping to remediate the pain caused by shingles inflicted nerve damage, especially PHN.

As I said in the last chapter, I didn't have much luck with scenar treatments. My own theory on this is that the doctor did not space the scenar applications close enough together to really make a difference. I was being scheduled for a single treatment once a week. It occurred to me that had I been exposed to this treatment twice a day for a full two weeks, the pain would have subsided and been remediated.

Another type of microcurrent pain relief protocol, Frequency-Specific Microcurrent treatment (or FSM), has had considerable success in helping to relieve the pain of postherpetic neuralgia. There are several high-profile clinics and practitioners that use this method, among them, the Cleveland Clinic.

Homeopathy

I didn't have the opportunity to try homeopathic remedies for shingles. However, Rhus tox is a homeopathic remedy that comes up, over and over again in discussions about protocols that have been known to speed up zoster remission - if it is taken at the outset of the disease. Here's a link that talks more about this and homeopathic remedies specific to shingles: http://www.britishhomeopathic.org/bha-charity/how-we-can-help/conditions-a-z/shingles-and-post-herpetic-neuralgia/

Homeopathic cocktails, in the hands of a trained and experienced practitioner, could be very valuable to some shingles sufferers. I spoke to at least one sufferer that said her doctor used homeopathy to bring about relief, and it apparently worked well for her. Below is a link to another website that talks in more depth about homeopathic remedies for shingles:

Alan Novarc

http://www.naturalnews.com/039071_shingles_homeopathic
_remedies_pain_relief.html

Chapter 9
What Worked

Again, my comments in this section have mostly to do with my own hands-on research and experience with these substances and protocols. Included, however, are protocols, substances, and regimens that showed great promise and were backed up by credible scientific sources.

There is no quick fix for shingles. This is a viral disease for which there is no patent cure. Resulting nerve damage heals slowly.   For this reason, it is important to utilize *all* available resources, including mainstream medicine's _ciclovir offerings. While the latter did not work for me, it may work for others. I did not experience side effects when using Famcyclovir.

Having said that, I did, in fact experience dramatic results when I began the regimen described below – a near immediate, fundamental shift in lessening the amount of suffering associated with the disease and an acceleration of the remediation process. The pain was more manageable, and there were clear indicators that the disease was in remission.

As I said earlier, there is a great deal of variability in the manifestation of shingles outbreaks. This lack of uniformity makes it more challenging to make sweeping claims about a single type of protocol working for everyone. So what I have done is first to include all of the elements of a protocol that I used personally to successfully find relief, and then include elements that are common to nearly all credible remediation protocols that I have discovered.

My outbreak was on my head, face and right eye. Yours might be on your torso or on your buttocks. Each of these types of outbreaks have their own particular issues. Some sufferers are more, some less sensitive to heat and cold, wind and touch, etc. The look, size and pattern of the lesions may be different. Some cases may be more intense than others. However, there is a commonality among them. For example, they are all herpes zoster infections that have had, as their pre-cursor either a pre-existing chickenpox infection somewhere in the history of the patient, or a recent exposure to the virus itself from someone else infected with the disease.

This baseline commonality makes it possible to share certain protocol elements across the spectrum of sufferers. Postherpetic neuralgia or PHN, the pain that lingers after the infection subsides, is caused by damage to the nerves that were infected by the virus – in all cases. The list below takes into consideration these commonalities.

Relief

In a previous chapter I talked about how important it was to find the right practitioner to work with right from the very outset of the disease. Unfortunately, I waited until the situation became unbearable, and even then I was only partially successful in finding someone who had real knowledge about remediation.

When I'd had enough, and was able to, I contacted an acquaintance who was a health products consultant to see if she had some advice. She suggested I email a natural medicine doctor friend to see if she was familiar with treating the infection.

I didn't expect much by email, but as a panicked sailor I was willing to try every option. The practitioner emailed me back the next day:

Take 10,000mcg B12 3x daily
Spray iWater [ionized water] on the affected area 10x a day.

That was it.

By this time I had already discovered the value of a water therapy (not iWater, but water from a garden hose or shower nozzle) in helping symptoms to subside (see *What Worked - Water Water Everywhere*).

At the time, I didn't know what the practitioner meant by iWater and was a little skeptical about purchasing any when I did find out. I know now that she meant ionized water and, at the time, I wasn't completely convinced about the efficacy of this substance, so I stuck with the water regimen that I was using.

Within a few hours of starting the B12 regimen, and already on the hose/shower water regimen that I will talk about in an upcoming chapter, I felt a significant shift in the disease, and it was at this time, precisely, that I could, for the first time in nearly a month, lay my head down on a pillow and sleep. I finally felt like I was on my way to healing. The above-mentioned practitioner's suggestions were invaluable in giving me the confidence to proceed with the water idea that I had stumbled upon and to move ahead with a natural protocol that included high-dose B12. Once again, this experience hinted at the importance of finding the right doctor to work with.

In hind sight, based on my first-hand experience and research, here's what I *should* have been doing for my shingles outbreak right from the very onset of the disease:

- **Find the right doctor/practitioner** to work with. (I should have done more to enlist friends and relatives to help with this; I went to mainstream doctors from the outset and was surprised to find how little they could help with shingles or PHN remediation).

- **High dose B12:** B12 injections, as directed, from a qualified practitioner or, 10,000mcg, single stage sublingual tablets of B12, 3x a day until symptoms subside (single-stage examples: Natural Factors methylcobalamin B12, 5,000mcg chewable or sublingual tablets; Costco's Kirkland brand methylcobalamin B12, 5,000mcg chewable or sublingual tablets, the latter being considerably less expensive). High doses of B12 are safe over extended periods of time for most people.

(If you are pregnant or have a medical condition besides shingles, see WebMDs comment about side effects here: http://www.webmd.com/vitamins-supplements/ingredientmono-926-vitamin%20b12.aspx?activeingredientid=926). Note that alcohol may interfere with B12 absorption.)

- **Acupuncture:** There is significant clinical evidence – double-blind studies – to indicate that acupuncture can be a significant aid in helping to bring about relatively quick relief from a shingles infection and its hideous symptoms. (http://www.healthcmi.com/Acupuncture-Continuing-Education-News/1314-acupuncture-beats-drugs-for-shingles-nerve-pain)

- **Vitamin B6:** take 50 to 75mg of B6 together with a good B-complex vitamin. Do not exceed 100mg B6 total dosage per day, as too much B6 can actually cause neuropathy and other problems. Monitor your dosages carefully, use higher dosages for the first 3 days of the outbreak. Continue lower dosages of B6 together with a good B-complex vitamin after initial high dosage stage.

- Injections of **adenosine monophosphate** by a qualified practitioner. There is clinical evidence suggesting that this works well for shingles infections, especially for pain during the PHN stages.

  (See: http://www.webmd.com/vitamins-supplements/ingredientmono-1067-adenosine.aspx?activeingredientid=1067&activeingredient name=adenosine)

- **Shower/garden hose treatments** 10 times a day, or as needed, cold or warm water depending on your comfort needs, especially for intermediate and later stages of shingles and PHN to help ease symptom discomfort and possibly help with pain remediation (see *What Worked - Water Water Everywhere*). Note: spraying aloe vera juice onto the affected area may possibly help in the very initial stages of the disease (see What Might Work).

- 2 capsules of **Moducare** three times per day for one week and 1 capsule three times per day thereafter for immune system optimization, typically from the outset of the disease (one capsule typically 20mg of sterols and 200mcg of sterolins).

- **400 IU of vitamin E** (mixed natural tocopherols) twice a day for three days and then 400 IU per day for optimal health (important note: if taking aspirin or other blood thinner, discuss high dose regimens with a doctor first).

- **Vitamin C injections**, as directed, by a qualified practitioner, or, 2,000 mg of buffered vitamin C every hour for three days, then 1,000-3,000 mg per day for maintenance (monitor for upset stomach or diarrhea - reduce dosage accordingly).

- **2,000mg of lysine** per day, with food, for the first three days during the disease period, and then 500mg for the next week. Use sporadically after a week, making good dietary choices your main source of lysine.

- **1,000mg monolaurin** capsules, 2x day from the outset of the disease until the malaise associated with the disease begins to subside.

- A good quality **lemon balm (*Melissa Officinalis*)** cream specifically for shingles may work well for topical application to the blistering. Clinical studies have shown the latter to be effective in supporting shingles remediation. Another topical cream choice that gets good reviews is Quantum lysine cream. Apply this to blisters, monitoring effectiveness. Calamine lotion may help to dry out blistering and relieve some of the itching.

Ah, but hind sight is always 20-20!

This is what I actually ended up doing (this was before I knew of the treatment options as listed above):

- B12 regimen (10,000 mcg sublingual, 3x a day)

- Hose/shower water regimen as needed (sometimes 10x a day)

- Vitamin C capsules, 3 to 4 grams a day

- 400IU vitamin E capsules 2x a day for four days and then once a day after that

- 500mg lysine capsules 2x a day

- 1,100mg monolaurin capsules, 2x a day

- Guided imagery healing session meditations, as noted in the *Natural Remedies* section of the booklet

This worked well for me, but I'm sure relief would have come much more quickly had I known about the what-I-*should*-have-done list above.

In my situation, I did not find a pain relief cream that worked for any length of time (see *Over the Counter Remedies* in the chapter on *What Didn't Work*). I didn't know about Quantum lysine cream or lemon balm cream until the PHN stage.

I didn't discover Moducare until later in the disease. Again, knowing what I know now, I would adhere to the first list above from the outset.

I did use the 'healing session' meditation regularly (see my explanation of this in *What Worked - The Mind Body Connection*).

Again, the guidance of the right practitioner, probably would have been very helpful in setting me on the right path from the beginning, avoiding weeks of lost work time, huge discomfort, and the frustration of having to wade through so many wrong leads. (See: *Finding the Right Doctor*)

Other potential remedies are interesting and may prove to be useful in some cases. I discuss these briefly in the chapter on *What Might Work* and provide the reader with some potentially useful links in the *Appendix* section.

Chapter 10
What Worked - Water Water Everywhere

Heat and Water

Heat will exacerbate the symptoms of some types of shingles and PHN episodes. It certainly did mine. I live in a warm climate. It was excruciating to be warm or hot, or to have my infected forehead and eye exposed to the sun, or anything warm, for that matter.

Fortunately, I like to swim and have access to a swimming beach nearby and a swimming pool about a 1/2 mile away. When I finally recognized that heat consistently made things worse, swimming sounded like a good idea. It was when I was showering off under a moderate-pressure shower with no shower head (vandals got the shower head) that I realized that the symptoms abated – almost completely for an hour and sometimes longer.

This got me thinking about using water to help alleviate the intensity of the burning, itching and pain, during the shingles infection period and beyond into the PHN period. I hooked up our garden hose with one of those on-off valves that can be purchased for the end of a hose. These are inexpensive and allow you to precisely control pressure with the little lever adjustment on the side of the valve. At first, I ran the water (adjusting the pressure and spray pattern carefully) from the hose across my forehead and lightly across the top, bottom and right side of my eye. No particular pattern or length of time, in the beginning.

I had read somewhere, maybe in a high school science class, that running water over certain substrates produced micro currents. After experiencing the scenar treatments (see section on scenar in *What Didn't Work*) I began to wonder if I wasn't setting up some kind of a microcurrent in the injured nerves by systematically running the water from the hose repeatedly over the area. This is essentially what actual microcurrent therapy does, but with much larger currents. I thought I would experiment with this idea. I had nothing to lose, I'd, so far, found nothing to help relieve the suffering, and by now, I was really and truly the scared sailor on a sinking ship.

This is the hose/shower water technique that eventually evolved, and that worked well for me:

- I used cold water (some may need warm water from a shower nozzle) Carefully adjust spray pattern and pressure of either garden hose or shower (I adjusted according to pain levels - what felt right at the time).

- A note about using an indoor shower for this technique: you may need to remove the spray end (unless it is adjustable for spray pattern) of your shower nozzle and just let the water from the end of the pipe stream onto the area. Better, attach a hose to the end of the pipe and direct the spray or stream precisely onto the affected area. If you've already got a hose-type shower, so much the better.

- Move the hose/shower water slowly, back and forth, over the affected area, using a straight, linear pattern, speeding up or slowing down the movement according to how it feels.

- Do this as many times as it takes to neutralize the pain and discomfort (for me, usually ten or twenty times - until I could no longer feel the pain in this area). You get the most benefit from this technique when you feel the pain subside while you are running the water over the area. Once it subsides, you have neutralized the pain and should feel a lot better, at least for a while.

- One hint about neutralizing the pain and discomfort while running water over the area: the tendency is to tense up when you run water over the sensitive area. I found that by focusing on, exhaling into and relaxing the area, and avoiding tensing up, that the pain dissipated much more quickly. It's almost as if you are exhaling the pain out of the wound. This little step turned out to be important.

- Again, I was careful to control the pressure precisely. Too much would have been counterproductive, not to mention very painful. Too little wouldn't have brought about the results I was looking for. As pain and sensitivity decreases, increase the pressure accordingly.

- At this point, I'd stop to see how it felt.

- Repeat the process as necessary. Sometimes I needed to do this procedure three or four times within a short period of time in order to get more lasting relief. So, complete a session and see how it feels. If there is still some discomfort, do it again.

- As time went on, the relief span lasted longer and longer.

What started out as a simple shower, turned out to be a very helpful regimen in providing some respite from the discomfort I was suffering.

Again, this worked for me. I would not have been able to do this in the very initial stages of the disease outbreak because I was just too sick to move. But, had I known, initially I could have tried spraying water from a plastic spray bottle onto the affected area, which is essentially what the naturopath, whom I mentioned earlier, suggested.

Also worth noting, and something I would have definitely tried, had I thought it was an option at that time, would be spraying or misting pure aloe vera juice on the infected area at the outset of the disease. One gallon containers of 99.8% pure aloe juice is widely available at Wal-Mart stores for a very reasonable price. Aloe juice in this form is as thin as water and would soak the skin very nicely without residue or unpleasant smells. In hind sight, I believe this might have helped when the infection first surfaced.

And while I'm on the topic of misting the infected area – I've alluded to this earlier in the book but it might be worth repeating here – there have been many reports of relief from shingles discomfort and the shrinking of lesions as a result of misting with apple cider vinegar, something I didn't try, but worth consideration.

Chapter 11
What Worked - The Mind Body Connection

I promised at the beginning of this book that I would share *everything* that I did to try and get better. Below might sound a bit flighty to some, but years of experience, and now science (see *Appendix*), has taught me that there is some merit to it. I found it quite helpful during my bout with shingles.

There is nothing flighty about the notion that your mind can influence your body's health and healing – negatively or positively. Concepts like psychosomatic healing/disease, placebo effect, benefit or harm of a doctor's bedside manner, are well established concepts, even in mainstream medicine. So much so, in fact, that a relatively new discipline within medical science is attempting to decipher how this all works. Psychoneuroimmunology (PNI) is a division of mainstream medical research that conducts studies on the mind/body – or neurological/physiological – effect.

(see: http://www.bbc.com/news/health-26191713)

The power of the placebo (mind/body) experience, for example, has been verified by studies at Harvard and Cambridge Universities and documented in a recently released film entitled The Power of the Placebo:

Best quality version:
http://www.dailymotion.com/video/x1z4iyq_e07-the-power-of-the-placebo_tv

The same documentary is also available in two parts on YouTube but at a very low quality:
https://www.youtube.com/watch?v=_v6nPcHgBXQ

I have been experimenting with mind/body healing ideas for about 10 years, seeing if I could create a healing environment when there was disease present. I found that the mind can accelerate the already inevitable natural process of healing. We are designed to heal and humans (and other living things) tend to experience disease/healing cycles regularly.

While healing is a natural phenomenon, natural healing is not a panacea in and of itself. The problem is in rate of healing. If we are made severely ill by a fast-spreading disease or blunt trauma, chances are that our natural healing tendencies will not serve us quickly enough to save our lives. This is where mainstream medicine shines. Often, quick intervention with the right protocol can stabilize a sick or injured person long enough for the healing process to do its work.

Because this is a separate subject unto itself, I won't go into detail here as to how to get the mind involved with healing. Instead I will share some key points and let the reader research on his or her own the salient details (see *Appendix*).

I start by getting comfortable in a chair or lying down in bed.

First, breathing.

Any mind/body healing session starts with breath. In yoga, exhaling into a difficult pose often helps the practitioner to achieve better results. Exhaling into pain while relaxing that area with the mind (really allowing that area to just 'drop to the floor' with relaxation) is the first step in getting one's mind completely focused on the area of concern. I usually inhale for four counts, hold the breath for six counts, and exhale for as long as my natural rhythm allows. The exhale is the main focus, imagining that the symptoms/disease are being carried out of the body on the breath. I try to maintain this image by not inhaling in the same spot that I just exhaled, so moving my head to one side on the next inhale.

Second, guided imagery.

As we've just seen, I use the image of the disease being carried away by the exhaling breath. There are lots of different images that are possible, or that can be used together. The trick is, to find one that resonates with you.

Third, how badly do you want to get better?

If you are angry or passionate enough about your recovery, this can be a tool to help with mind/body healing session. Exhale into the disease/pain and know to the depth of your being you want to get better. Some say that downright anger, in this case, can be an asset.

Forth, movement.

When you are doing one of these healing sessions, you need your mind's full attention. I find that doing this in bed allows me to do a mild convulse, as it were, beginning from the abdomen, to bring my mind back fully to the healing process. I sync this movement with my heartbeat and let the motion gently move through my body.

Fifth, sound.

Again, to help focus and give some dimension to the process, I will occasionally do a low OM-like sound, similar to that used in some meditations. Again, this helps with focus and also adds another dimension to the process.

During my recovery period, I used this healing session method to help speed remediation. It was another tool in the quiver and I felt it was very useful.

One cautionary note: when you start getting good at this, you can create heat in the area of concern. Sometimes this is good, and sometimes not. For the purposes of this booklet, if you are trying, with this technique, to heal the neuralgic pain or sensation that may be signaling the *potential onset* of a herpes zoster infection, and you are creating heat in that location, stop, because you may actually precipitate a shingles outbreak. Heat seems to create an ideal environment for the onset of some versions of shingles. I learned this the hard way (see *Why Me? Heat as a precursor to an imminent outbreak*) – another reason to pay close attention to what your body is trying to tell you.

Chapter 12
What Worked - Exercise?

When I got to a point in the disease cycle where I could move around again, I started going for walks, swimming, doing yoga, and an exercise called chi gung. Whatever I could comfortably manage at the time. I found this to be important from two standpoints: firstly, getting the circulation going so that the disease area is constantly exposed to everything the immune system has to offer for remediation. Secondly, the distraction helps alleviate some of the discomfort.

Yoga

I have found that yoga, particularly, with its breathing component, gentle stretching, and focus on relaxation was particularly helpful. If you are new to yoga, it might pay to invest in a Hatha Yoga instructional video, or check out some of the yoga classes on YouTube. I do a gentle yoga routine that takes about 30 minutes or so to complete. The effect, when done correctly, is better than medications.

Chi gung

A popular exercise in China and increasingly throughout the rest of the world, chi gung, like yoga, is a gentle exercise that incorporates breathing, movement, some stretching, and meditation. In addition to its physical and mental benefits, Chi gung is meant to help circulate your chi, or core life-force energy. While, to a westerner, this may sound a bit strange, there are millions of chi gung adepts who use this concept to enhance their health, sense of wellbeing, and longevity. You do not have to be athletic or someone who regularly meditates to practice chi gung. Any body type is fine, and any conditioning is okay. There are some good chi gung training videos on YouTube for beginners through intermediates.

Tai chi

Across the board, the exercise most recommended for PHN sufferers is tai chi. While tai chi's benefits are similar to chi gung, tai chi is, when properly mastered, an advanced exercise form that requires training from a qualified instructor. There are 108 different movements in yang style tai chi, the most popular form, that need to be stored in your muscle memory. If you are not a tai chi adept when you are infected with shingles, now would not be the time to take up this exercise form. This may be something to put on your bucket list after you are fully recovered.

I have been doing tai chi for over 25 years. It has been very helpful during the PHN stages of the disease. However, I was not able to do the exercise during the shingles infection itself. Blind in one eye, balance compromised, weak and tired, I did not feel up to a tai chi session. Chi gung was the better option, as soon as I could muster the energy.

Swimming

I can't say enough about this exercise form for shingles and PHN sufferers. I did it as much as I could, starting in the intermediate stages of my shingles infection, right through the PHN stages. In a pool, lake or ocean, the water buoys you up, and suspends the effects of gravity while you move through the water in whatever way your skill level allows. The exercise involves proper breathing, coordination, and light to moderate exertion. And the nice cool shower afterwards, for me, was pure heaven!

Jogging

I tried jogging during the intermediate stages of the infection itself. This was not fun. Jogging can deplete energy quickly, and the irritation of clothing over a torso-based shingles infection, or the debilitating pain and potential lack of balance in those suffering with a face, head, or eye infection makes this a difficult trick. After having tried it, I don't recommend it until later in the PHN stages. Even then, monitor for the benefits.

Bicycling

I bicycled right from the intermediate stages of the infection right on through the PHN stage. Bicycling worked okay for me, with some caveats. I did have to be more careful than usual because of the loss of sight in my right eye and the balance issues. But with focused care, a bike ride can help keep your cardio up a bit and provide you with much needed exercise without excess exertion.

Light Calisthenics

A regimen of pushups, sit ups, pull ups/chin ups, etc., might best be left for after the shingles infection. I do these exercises when I am healthy. Many sufferers will not have the strength or the will to dive into this kind of regimen. There is also the issue of rest. If I had to choose between calisthenics and rest during the shingles disease period, I'd choose rest. During the PHN period, I did start to do some light calisthenics again, and they were mildly beneficial.

Light weights and machine exercises

Again, as with calisthenics, this might be something better left for the post shingles stage. If you are suffering from PHN, I'm not sure how much this would actually help. I haven't tried this, so I can't say for sure. One rule of thumb though, if you are going to get back into a weight training and machine exercise routine, start out light and see how it feels. Diving right back in, full bore, may set you back in your remission process.

The benefits of movement

Some form of light exertion, movement, and activity is important to healthy remission. There is no need to be an athlete or to even be athletically inclined. Just getting out

Alan Novarc

and taking a walk is beneficial – moving around, when possible, seems to help support faster healing, especially when done out-of-doors.

Chapter 13
Being Proactive - Preventative Care

⊥here is nothing that you can do about your history with chickenpox. Just know that you could be a candidate for a shingles infection if you've had chickenpox somewhere in your past. A possibility too, however small, is contracting shingles as a result of exposure to someone else with the disease.

What you *can* do to reduce the possibility of an infection is to monitor your diet with an eye towards lysine levels and supplementing as needed, keeping your stress levels under control, and making sure you're getting enough B-complex, C, and E. Your single best protection is a robust, healthy immune system, so supplementation that boosts immune efficiency, for example, plant sterols and sterolins, might be a solid component to a good plan.

Warning signs of an imminent shingles outbreak

The biggest mistake I made was not realizing that the pain I was experiencing over and around my right eye, for months, had the potential to be ground zero for a zoster attack. Some people say they experience an 'unusual sensation' in the area that will experience the infection. Paying attention to persistent neuralgic pain, or sensations, especially around the eyes, forehead, and anywhere on the torso will allow for an early assault on the disease. In my case, heat was a significant antagonizer, and it was heat applied directly to the painful area that was the final trigger in the outbreak on my forehead and around my right eye (see the section on *What Worked - The Mind/Body Connection*, bottom of the page beginning with: *One cautionary note*).

In my case, treating the painful area - before an outbreak - with cold compresses, may have been a strategy I could have employed to help stop or delay the onset. Of course, this is hind sight. However, in most cases where there is an imminent shingles outbreak, immediately upping dosages of lysine and monolaurin, starting on Moducare capsules, and upping doses of vitamin C, E, and B12 (see *What Worked*), and perhaps beginning a regimen of made-for-shingles homeopathic substances.

(For more information about sterols and sterolins see: http://www.naturalnews.com/039071_shingles_homeopathic _remedies_pain_relief.html)

In my case, the lysine supplements would have been particularly helpful because of my extremely high arginine levels prior to the infection. This arginine rich environment may have played a significant role in creating a lysine deficient/arginine prolific situation - a precursor for herpes zoster migration and outbreak. Knowing what I know now,

I would have also considered beginning the protocol noted in the first list in the *What Worked* section of the booklet.

Everyone I spoke to who had a shingles outbreak said they had been under stress. Everyone, no exceptions. All felt that stress was a prerequisite to shingles. This was certainly true in my case. The warning signs of shingles may also be a warning sign about over-the-top stress.

What about the herpes zoster vaccination?

There are claims being made that the number of shingles cases in the U.S. has dropped dramatically since the inception of Merck corporation's Zostavax. Unfortunately, the facts present too many contradictions.

First of all, anyone doing research on the subject will not fail to notice the legion of zoster infection sufferers who actually had a shingles vaccine.

Secondly, while Merck, upon releasing Zostavax, wanted us to believe that the drug would be at least 70% - 90% effective, new evidence now suggests something closer to 18% - 51% effective, depending on how old you are. Credibility is an issue. There are just too many conflicts in the information being presented to the public about Zostavax, with too many testimonials to non-beneficial reactions to the drug.

The choice, ultimately, is in the hands of the individual. One thing is for certain, if there is no history of chickenpox in your background, you may want to think very carefully before spending the $200, or so, on a shingles vaccination.

A cautionary word about the potentially dangerous preliminary stages of a shingles outbreak

It is very important to be on high alert, so to speak, when you first come down with a shingles infection, especially when the eye or eyes are involved. This is the time, when you least feel like it, to really be aware of what you need in any given moment. By all means, go to a doctor, immediately, and take the prescription drug on offer. Start a supplement protocol immediately that will support shingles remediation. Immediately get help with finding a practitioner who is familiar with alternative protocols for shingles relief. Make sure you get enough to eat, that you are having regular bowl movements, and that you do not put yourself in a situation where you are exposed to other potential infections or mishaps. When you have shingles on the face, head and in the eye, it is possible to experience balance problems which may cause serious falls. Injuries during this initial period could be very dangerous. If ever there was a time to take full charge of yourself, it would be during the initial outbreak period. Cascading failure caused by additional infections or injuries could make the shingles experience much more dangerous than it needs to be.

I hope that the reader was able to benefit from my booklet by, at the very least, helping to focus efforts and resources efficiently. If you are a shingles sufferer, I wish you a speedy recovery and a happy and healthy life!

Appendix

In this section, I have provided the reader with some additional links for further research. This is by no means a definitive list. The reader is encouraged to use key words to do more in-depth research on the Internet.

General overview: The Herpes Zoster Infection (About Shingles)

A detailed overview of the shingles infection; Health Guide, the New York Times:
http://www.nytimes.com/health/guides/disease/herpes-zoster/print.html

Herpes Zoster; University of Maryland:
http://umm.edu/health/medical/reports/articles/shingles-and-chickenpox-varicellazoster-virus

Herpes Zoster; Winchester Hospital:
http://www.winchesterhospital.org/health-library/article?id=21722

In depth explanation of the herpes zoster virus and infection: Wikipedia:
https://en.wikipedia.org/wiki/Shingles

The Zostervax shingles vaccine

From the Food and Drug Administration:
http://www.fda.gov/BiologicsBloodVaccines/Vaccines/QuestionsaboutVaccines/ucm070418.htm

Zostervax controversy:
http://www.thehealthyhomeeconomist.com/the-shingles-vaccine-help-or-hype/

Homeopathic suggestions for remediation:

Shingles and post-herpetic neuralgia; British Homeopathic Association:

http://www.britishhomeopathic.org/bha-charity/how-we-can-help/conditions-a-z/shingles-and-post-herpetic-neuralgia/

Herpes Zoster Symptoms - Homeopathic Relief; Natural News:
http://www.naturalnews.com/039071_shingles_homeopathic_remedies_pain_relief.html

Homeopathic medicine for shingles; Vitality Magazine:
http://vitalitymagazine.com/article/homeopathic-medicine-for-shingles-herpes-zoster/

Naturopathic shingles relief protocols

Properly trained, credible naturopathic and alternative practitioners are no strangers to the shingles infection. Most patients are finding that their regular doctor doesn't have a cure for shingles or PHN, or the pain and discomfort associated with this disease. As a result, many are turning to alternative practitioners for help.

Shingles remediation, naturally; Health Solutions:
http://healthyimmunity.com/qanda/31-Shingles.asp

Five natural treatments for shingles; Healthline:
http://www.healthline.com/health-slideshow/shingles-natural-treatment

Lysine and the shingles infection

The role of lysine deficiency as one predeterminate for a shingles outbreak is becoming better understood as studies begin to define the interrelationship of lysine and arginine. It is important to understand that arginine is not a bad substance,

but rather one that is kept in balance. Arginine is essential to
the repair of peripheral neuropathy (PHN, and so a proper
balance of the two substances is especially meaningful to post
shingles PHN sufferers.

University of Maryland on Lysine:
http://umm.edu/health/medical/altmed/supplement/lysine

Lysine and arginine and shingles; LiveStrong Magazine:
http://www.livestrong.com/article/274365-l-lysine-and-shingles/

More about Monolaurin

Antiviral actions of monolaurin; Advanced Healing:
http://www.advancedhealing.com/antiviral-antibacterial-actions-of-
monolaurin-and-lauric-acid/

User reviews of monolaurin; WebMD:
http://www.webmd.com/vitamins-supplements/ingredientreview-
1149-MONOLAURIN

**Plant sterols and sterolins (Moducare); Immune system
health:**

Sterol and sterolin role in immune system modulation;
National Institute of Health:
http://www.ncbi.nlm.nih.gov/pubmed/10383481
Plant sterols and sterolins for herpes outbreaks; Alive
Magazine:

http://www.alive.com/health/plant-sterols-and-sterolins/

Vitamin C and shingles

Intravenous C used in the treatment of shingles; National
Institute of Health:
http://www.ncbi.nlm.nih.gov/pubmed/22460093

High dose intravenous vitamin C for the treatment of shingles;
Riordan Clinic:
 https://riordanclinic.org/2014/02/high-dose-intravenous-vitamin-c-
as-a-successful-treatment-of-viral-infections/

High dose vitamin B12 regimen

Article about shingles, see section on the effectiveness of high
dose B12 remediation; ZHealthInfo:
http://www.zhealthinfo.com/shingles.htm

Vitamin B12 and Herpes Zoster Infections; Whole Health
Insider:
http://www.wholehealthinsider.com/immune-system/surviving-
shingles/

High dose vitamin E

Supplement support for shingles; Holistic-Online:
http://www.holistic-
online.com/remedies/Shingles/shingles_vitamin.htm

Alternative remedies for shingles - vitamin E treatment;
HomeopathyWorldCommunity:
http://www.homeopathyworldcommunity.com/forum/topics/shingles
-vitamins-and

Melissa Officinalis, or Lemon Balm

Melissa Officinalis effectiveness relating to herpes infections;
National Institutes of Health:
http://www.ncbi.nlm.nih.gov/pubmed/18693101

Applying melissa officinalis to herpes infections; LiveStrong:
http://www.livestrong.com/article/105847-use-lemon-balm-herpes/

Adenosine monophosphate injections

Adenosine Monophosphate overview; WebMD:
http://www.webmd.com/vitamins-supplements/ingredientmono-1067-adenosine.aspx?activeingredientid=1067&activeingredientname=adenosine

Adenosine Monophosphate overview; therapy-EPNet:
http://therapy.epnet.com/nat/GetContent.asp?chunkiid=40003

Capsicum

Topical capsicum application for neuralgic pain; The National Institute of Health:
http://www.ncbi.nlm.nih.gov/pmc/articles/PMC3169333/

Capsicum overview; WebMD:
http://www.webmd.com/vitamins-supplements/ingredientmono-945-capsicum.aspx?activeingredientid=945&activeingredientname=capsicum

Mind/body psychosomatic responses

There is a great deal of information on the web on this subject, some of it based in science, and some based on subjective observation. Below I list links to Harvard and Cambridge studies on the subject.

BBC article, "Medicine in our Minds":
http://www.bbc.com/news/health-26191713

BBC Documentary, "The Power of the Placebo" (best quality version):
http://www.dailymotion.com/video/x1z4iyq_e07-the-power-of-the-placebo_tv

The same documentary is also available in two parts on YouTube but at a very low quality:
https://www.youtube.com/watch?v=_v6nPcHgBXQ

Acupuncture/Acupressure

How acupuncture can help during a shingles infection: BritishAcupunctureCouncil:
http://www.acupuncture.org.uk/a-to-z-of-conditions/a-to-z-of-conditions/herpes.html

Treating shingles pain with acupuncture; HealthCMI:
http://www.healthcmi.com/Acupuncture-Continuing-Education-News/1314-acupuncture-beats-drugs-for-shingles-nerve-pain

Benefits of exercise to help with the healing process

Exercise and shingles; LiveStrong:
http://www.livestrong.com/article/313649-should-you-exercise-with-shingles/
Exercise and shingles, the ups and downs; DailyStrength:
https://www.dailystrength.org/group/shingles/discussion/3-1350188074-85565773030b8833a

www.ingramcontent.com/pod-product-compliance
Lightning Source LLC
Chambersburg PA
CBHW020334290526
45785CB00005B/2007